Landmarks for Peripheral Nerve Blocks

Upper and Lower Extremities

SECOND EDITION

Didier A. Sciard, M.D.

Maria E. Matuszczak, M.D.

Associate Professors
Department of Anesthesiology
The University of Texas–Houston Medical School
Houston, Texas

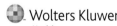
Wolters Kluwer | Lippincott Williams & Wilkins
Health

Philadelphia · Baltimore · New York · London
Buenos Aires · Hong Kong · Sydney · Tokyo

AUTHOR CONSIDERATIONS

This pocket book is not designed to replace a regular atlas or textbook of regional anesthesia but may be carried by any anesthesiologist who wants to refresh his or her knowledge quickly.

The focus is on landmarks, some anatomic considerations, and tips.

Regional anesthesia can be used as the sole anesthetic technique or can be combined with general anesthesia for postoperative pain management.

In any case this technique must be performed for the patient's benefit so as to achieve the best and safest surgical conditions.

A new scientific truth does not triumph because it convinces its opponents, making them see the light, but rather because its opponents eventually die and a new generation grows up that is familiar with it.

Max Planck (1858–1947)

Contributing author: **Nicholas Lam, M.D.**
Assistant Professor
Department of Anesthesiology
The University of Texas–Houston Medical School
Houston, Texas

Illustrator: **Alexandre Matuszczak**

Acquisitions Editor: Brian Brown
Managing Editor: Nicole T. Dernoski
Project Manager: Fran Gunning
Manufacturing Manager: Ben Rivera
Marketing Manager: Angela Panetta
Design Coordinator: Stephen Druding
Production Services: International Typesetting and Composition

© 2008 by Lippincott Williams & Wilkins, a Wolters Kluwer business
530 Walnut Street
Philadelphia, PA 19106
LWW.com

Library of Congress Cataloging-in-Publication Data

Sciard, Didier A.
  Landmarks for peripheral nerve blocks : upper and lower extremities /
Didier A. Sciard, Maria E. Matuszczak ; contributing author, Nicholas Lam ;
illustrator, Alexandre Matuszczak.—2nd ed.
    p. ; cm.
  ISBN-13: 978-0-7817-8752-9
  ISBN-10: 0-7817-8752-1
  1. Nerve block—Handbooks, manuals, etc. I. Matuszczak, Maria E. II. Lam,
Nicholas. III. Title.
  [DNLM: 1. Nerve Block—methods—Handbooks. 2. Lower
Extremity—Handbooks. 3. Peripheral Nerves—anatomy & histology—Handbooks.
4. Upper Extremity—Handbooks. WO 231 S416L 2008]
  RD84.S46 2008
  617.4'8—dc22

                                                            2007029223

CONTENTS

PRINCIPLES OF NEUROSTIMULATION

Appropriate Location and Equipment

- Room equipped with standard ASA monitors
- Immediate access to resuscitative drugs and equipment
- Equipment checked
- Neurostimulators able to deliver a current of up to 5-mA intensity, frequency of 1 or 2 Hz (1 or 2 impulses per second), impulse duration of 0.1 to 1 msec (0.1 to 0.3 msec for a motor nerve stimulation and 1 msec for a sensory nerve stimulation)
- Insulated needles of 1, 2, 4, and 6 inches (2.5, 5, 10, and 15 cm)
- Catheter sets with 2-, 4-, and 6-inch (5-, 10-, and 15-cm) introducer needles

Technique

- Check nerve stimulator and connecting cables for their proper function.
- Skin prep and local infiltrate for needle insertion.
- Minimal distance between skin electrode and needle.
- After skin puncture, gradually increase the intensity up to 1.5 mA at 0.3 msec.
- Search in 3 axes (see picture on page x).
- As soon as the first twitch is obtained, impulse duration (msec) should be decreased to 0.1 msec. Then intensity (mA) is slowly decreased while approaching the nerve to a minimal stimulation intensity of 0.5 to 0.3 mA.
- Aspirate for blood.
- Loss of motor response after injection of 1 mL of local anesthetic and return of the motor response when intensity is increased.
- No resistance or pain during injection.
- Slow and fragmented injection.

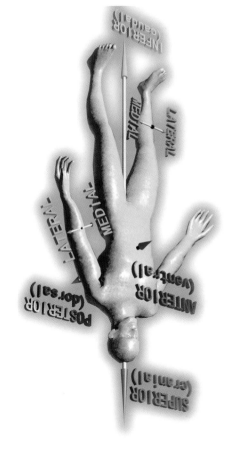

DEFINITIONS

- **Superior (or cranial):** toward the head.
- **Inferior (or caudal):** toward the feet.
- **Anterior (or ventral):** toward the front of the body.
- **Posterior (or dorsal):** toward the back of the body.
- **Medial:** toward the median plane.
- **Lateral:** away from the median plane.
- **Supination:** rotation of the radius around its long axis so that the palm faces anteriorly.
- **Pronation:** rotation of the radius around its long axis so that the palm faces posteriorly.
- **Adduction:** moving toward the median plane.
- **Abduction:** moving away from the median plane.

Upper Extremity Landmarks

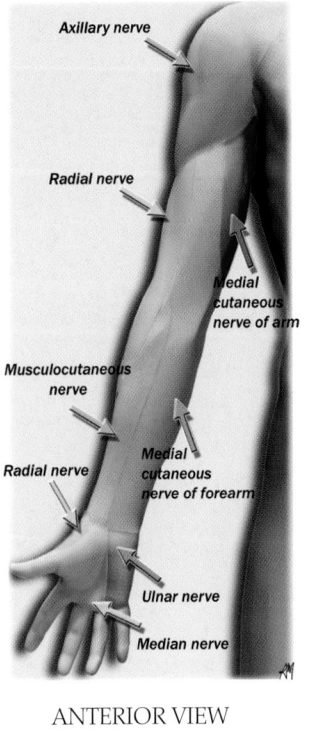

POSTERIOR VIEW

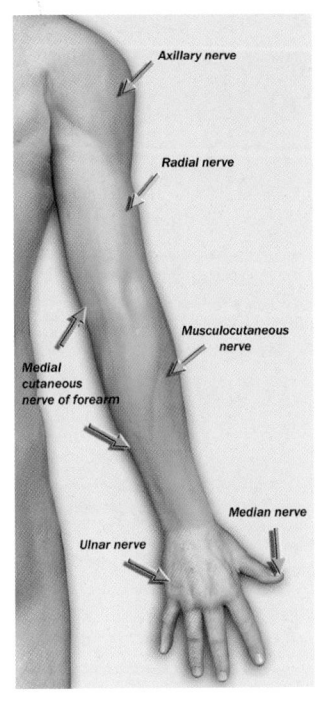

ANTERIOR VIEW

DERMATOMES

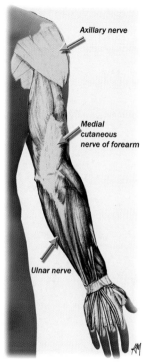

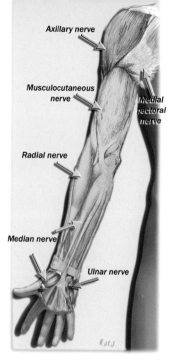

ANTERIOR VIEW

MYOTOMES

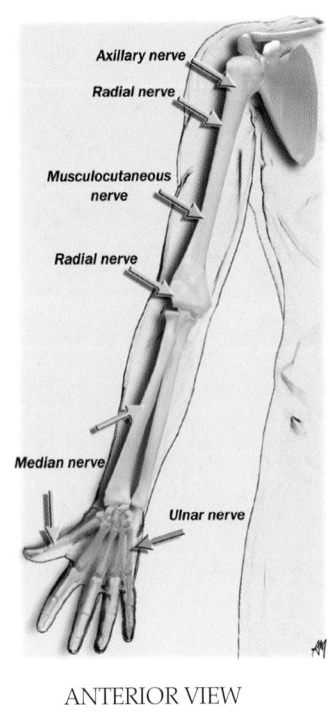

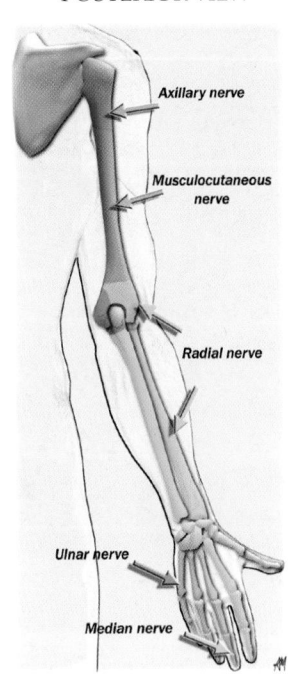

POSTERIOR VIEW

Axillary nerve

Radial nerve

Musculocutaneous
nerve

Radial nerve

Median nerve

Ulnar nerve

ANTERIOR VIEW

Axillary nerve

Musculocutaneous
nerve

Radial nerve

Ulnar nerve

Median nerve

OSTEOTOMES

BRACHIAL PLEXUS BLOCK

- Formed from anterior primary rami of C5-T1.
- 5 roots, 3 trunks, 3 cords, 5 nerves.
- 3 trunks: upper (C5, C6), middle (C7), and lower (C8, T1) in the interscalene space, anterior to scalenus medius and posterior to scalenus anterior.
- The trunks pass over the lateral border of the first rib and under the clavicle; each trunk (superior, middle, and inferior) divides into anterior and posterior branches. The branches reunite to form cords.
- 3 cords around the axillary artery:
  - Lateral cord: lateral portion of the median nerve and musculocutaneous nerve.
  - Medial cord: medial portion of the median nerve, ulnar nerve, medial cutaneous nerve of the forearm, and medial cutaneous nerve of the arm.
  - Posterior cord: axillary and radial nerves.

AXILLARY

A
- Cervical C5, C6.
- Posterior to the third part of axillary artery.
- Run laterally to the surgical neck of the humerus.
- Posterior branch gives off the upper lateral nerve of the arm.

S
- Cutaneous innervation of the shoulder.
- Deltoid.
- Shoulder joint.

N
- Contraction of the deltoid.

A Anatomy **S** Surgical field **N** Neurostimulation

MUSCULOCUTANEOUS

A • Cervical C5, C6.

S • Cutaneous innervation of the lateral part of the forearm.
• Ventral musculature of the arm.

N • Flexion of the forearm by contraction of the biceps (long and short head).
• Possible confusion with a radial stimulation. The contraction of the supinator and brachioradialis muscles innervated by the radial gives a *flexion and supination* of the forearm.

A Anatomy **S** Surgical field **N** Neurostimulation

RADIAL

A
- Cervical C6, C8.
- Posterior to the axillary and brachial arteries.
- Run with the profunda brachii artery between the long and medial heads of triceps.
- Before leaving the axilla, the radial nerve gives the posterior cutaneous nerve of arm that innervates the posterior upper arm skin.
- The posterior cutaneous nerve of forearm innerves the posterior forearm skin.
- The deep radial branch innerves the forearm musculature and posterior part of carpal bones.
- The superficial radial nerve passes over the tendons of the snuff box and terminates as cutaneous branches to the dorsum of the hand.

S
- Cutaneous innervation of the posterior part of the arm, forearm, and posterolateral part of the hand.
- Extensor muscles (dorsal musculature in the upper extremity below the shoulder).
- Radioulnar joint and wrist joint.

N
- Extension and supination of forearm.
- Extension of the wrist and the fingers.
- Abduction and extension of the thumb.

A Anatomy **S** Surgical field **N** Neurostimulation

MEDIAN

A • Cervical C6, thoracic T1.
- The median nerve lies lateral to the axillary artery and then lateral to the brachial artery before crossing the artery at the level of the midhumerus.
- Gives branch to elbow joint (superior portion of the radioulnar joint): capitulum of humerus, radial head, and epitrochlea of humerus.
- Gives branch to pronator muscles at level of forearm (one of the terminal branches is the anterior interosseous n.).
  - Arises just below the two heads of pronator teres m.
  - Contraction of flexor digitorum superficialis = flexion of proximal interphalangeal (IP) joints and secondary metacarpophalangeal (MCP) joints and wrist.

- Contraction of flexor digitorum profundus *(60% to 70% median and 30% to 40% ulnar)* = flexion of distal IP joints and secondary flexion of proximal IP and MCP joints and wrist.

S
- Elbow joint (radioulnar joint).
- Cutaneous innervation of the lateral palmar skin.
- Ventral musculature of the forearm (flexor and pronator muscles).
- Wrist and lower radioulnar joint (sensory supply to the anterior part of carpal bones).

N
- Flexion of the fingers and wrist.
- Pronation of the wrist.
- Opposition of the thumb (adductor pollicis brevis and opponens pollicis).

A Anatomy **S** Surgical field **N** Neurostimulation

Martin and Gruber Anastomosis

Median and ulnar anastomosis at forearm.

Present in 20% of patients.

Median and ulnar stimulations give the same flexion of the digits (flexion of the last 2 digits and adduction of the thumb) but *adduction and flexion of the wrist* are exclusively obtained with ulnar stimulation (no anastomosis with flexor carpi ulnaris).

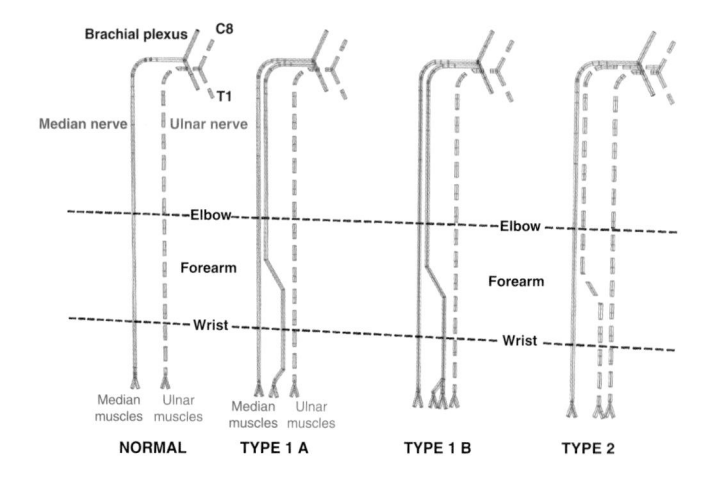

ULNAR

A
- Cervical C8, thoracic T1.
- Medial to the axillary and brachial arteries.
- Gives a branch to *elbow joint*: olecranon and medial epicondyle of humerus.
- Divides into terminal branches at the pisiform bone.
- Dorsal cutaneous branch arises 5 cm proximal to the wrist; passes deep to flexor carpi ulnaris.

S
- Cutaneous innervation of the medial part of the hand.
- Ventral musculature of the hand.
- Deep terminal branch: wrist joint, interossei, lumbricals, adductor pollicis, flexor pollicis brevis.

N
- Adduction of the thumb and little finger.
- Prehension by the little finger and thumb.
- Adduction and supination of the wrist.
- Martin and Gruber anastomosis: see median.

Tips:

- Elbow joint innervation = radial, median, and ulnar.
- Wrist joint innervation = radial (posterior interosseous), median, and ulnar (deep terminal branch).
- Medial cutaneous nerve of arm and forearm arise from the medial cord (C8-T1 roots).

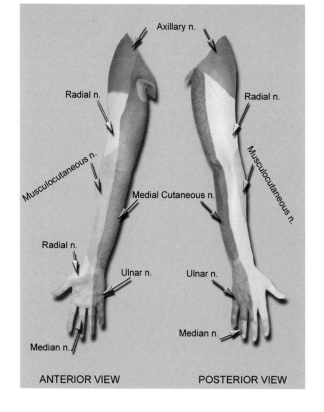

ANTERIOR VIEW

POSTERIOR VIEW

UPPER EXTREMITY: DERMATOMES

INTERSCALENE APPROACH

Patient position: Supine, head turned slightly to the opposite side.

Landmarks:
- Line along the lateral border of the clavicular head of the sternocleidomastoid muscle (SCM).
- Line between the thyroid and cricoid cartilages (C5-C6).
- Intersection of these 2 lines.

Tips:
- 1- or 2-inch needle.
- The clavicular head of the SCM is easily identified by asking the patient to lift up his or her head.
- The puncture point is lateral and posterior to the SCM and the external jugular vein, which overlies the SCM. The brachial plexus lies between the anterior and middle parts of the

scalene muscle, posterior and lateral to the lateral border of the clavicular head of the SCM.

- Needle is directed caudal, posterior, and medial with a 45-degree angle.
- If the needle tip is inserted *too posterior*, a *contraction* of the levator scapulae muscle by stimulation of the dorsal scapular nerve can be confused with a deltoid contraction. Placing one hand over the scapula can make a differential.
- *Contraction of the diaphragm* by stimulation of the phrenic n., which runs over the lateral border of scalenus anterior m. behind the prevertebral fascia, means that the needle tip is inserted *too anteriorly.*
- The roots C8 and T1 (median and ulnar nerves) are partially blocked or not blocked with this approach.
- A catheter can be inserted for a continuous interscalene block.
- *Side effects*: Horner's syndrome (stellate ganglion block), hoarse voice (recurrent laryngeal nerve), 100% ipsilateral paralysis of the diaphragm (phrenic nerve).

- *Can occur:*

Minor = difficulty in swallowing (recurrent laryngeal nerve).

Major = total spinal anesthesia, vertebral artery injection.

A test dose (3 to 5 mL) and a slow fragmented injection (10 mL/30 sec) are essential.

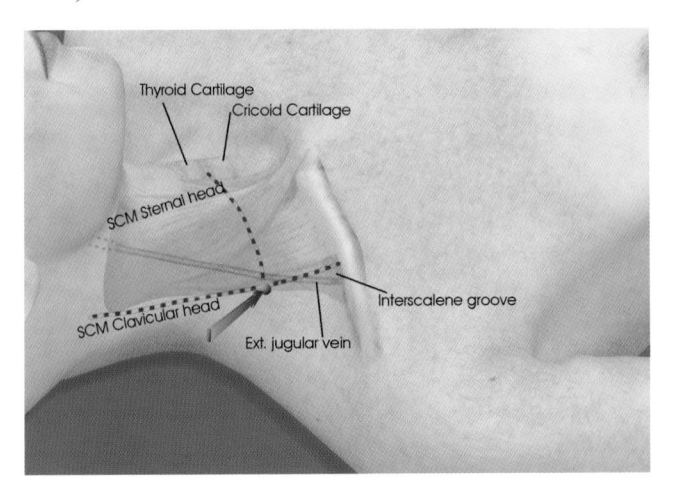

INTERSCALENE APPROACH

SUPRACLAVICULAR APPROACH

Patient position: Supine, limb along the body or forearm flexed on the trunk.

Landmarks:
- Line along the lateral border of the clavicular head of the SCM.
- Line along the clavicle.
- Intersection of these two lines.
- Subclavian artery in the supraclavicular fossa.

Tips:
- 2-inch needle (plexus is located at a depth of 2 to 4 cm).

  Classic approach:
- Point of needle insertion is posterior and lateral to the subclavian artery.
- Position of needle is parallel to the neck and directed toward the first rib.

Plumb bob technique:

- Point of needle insertion is posterior and lateral to the SCM at its insertion on the clavicle.
- Position of needle is perpendicular to the neck and directed with a 30-degree angle in the caudal direction.
- *Nerve stimulation resulting in movements of the hand is essential* (radial, median, or ulnar).
- A contraction of the arm muscles is not sufficient.
- *Can occur:* pneumothorax, if needle is directed too medial and too posterior.

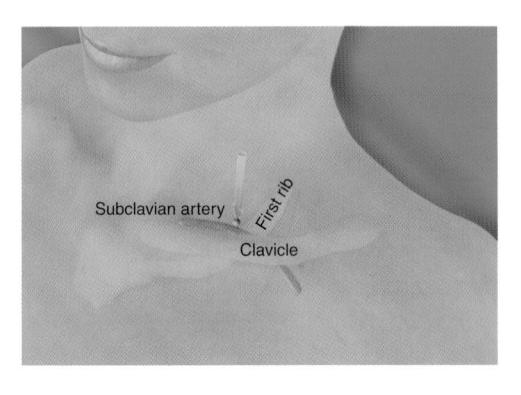

SUPRACLAVICULAR APPROACH

INFRACLAVICULAR APPROACH

Patient position: Supine, limb along the body or forearm flexed on the trunk.

Vertical Infraclavicular Approach

Landmarks:
- Midpoint of a line between ventral border of acromion of the scapula (lateral landmark) and fossa jugularis (medial landmark).

Tips:
- Just below or 1 cm caudal to the clavicle.
- *Strictly vertical* to the supine position of the patient.
- *Can occur:* pneumothorax, if needle directed too medial and deeper than 6 cm.

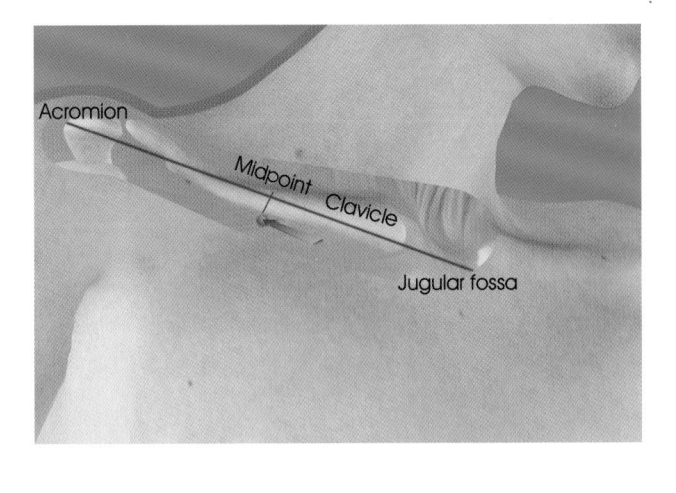

VERTICAL INFRACLAVICULAR APPROACH

Paracoracoid Approach

Landmarks:
- Ventral border of the coracoid process (fingertip on the tip of the coracoid process).
- 2 cm caudal and 2 cm medial, needle perpendicular to the skin or directed slightly cephalad.

Tips:

- 2- to 4-inch needle (4- to 6-cm depth depending on the needle's angle).
- *Obtaining a movement of the hand is essential* (radial, median, or ulnar).
- A musculocutaneous stimulation (biceps contraction) indicates an approach of the lateral part of the plexus (lateral cord). The needle must be directed more medially to obtain a median stimulation and posteriorly to obtain a radial stimulation (posterior cord).
- A multistimulation technique (lateral and posterior cord) increases the success rate of this block.
- A catheter can be inserted for a continuous infraclavicular block.

PARACORACOID APPROACH

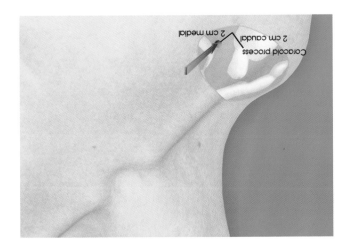

Coracoid process
2 cm caudal
2 cm medial

AXILLARY APPROACH

Patient position: Supine, arm abducted 90 degrees and rotated externally.

Landmarks:
- Lateral border of the pectoralis major.
- Axillary crease.
- Brachial artery.

Tips:

Single stimulation:
- Brachial artery is palpated high in the axilla crease.
- The needle is inserted directly above the artery, pointing almost parallel to the artery in a proximal direction with a 30- to 45-degree angle to the skin. A median, ulnar, or radial stimulation is elicited. (Do not accept a musculocutaneous stimulation.)
- A separate injection for the musculocutaneous nerve (see below) is advised.

- Slow and fragmented injection of the total dose of the local anesthetic solution with frequent aspiration.

Multistimulation:

- The needle is inserted directly above the artery, pointing to the artery in a proximal and medial direction at a 30- to 45-degree angle to the skin. A median stimulation is elicited (15 mL of local anesthetic).

- Above the artery and anterior into the coraco-brachialis muscle a musculocutaneous stimulation is elicited (5 mL of local anesthetic).

- Then the needle is inserted directly below the artery, pointing to the artery in a proximal and lateral direction at a 30- to 45-degree angle to the skin. A radial or ulnar (more superficial) stimulation is elicited (15 mL of local anesthetic).

- Anterior and posterior subcutaneous ring infiltration on the inner aspect of the axilla for the cutaneous nerves of the arm.

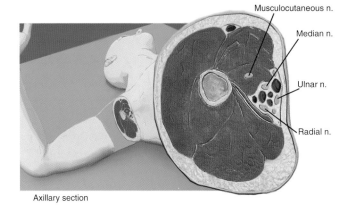

Musculocutaneous n.
Median n.
Ulnar n.
Radial n.

Axillary section

AXILLARY APPROACH

HUMERAL CANAL APPROACH

Patient position: Supine, arm abducted 90 degrees and rotated externally.

Landmark: Proximal third part of the arm.

MEDIAN

Landmark: Above the brachial artery on the inner arm.

Tips:
- Large nerve, very superficial, can be felt under the skin.
- To avoid penetrating the nerve, the needle is inserted parallel to the skin and then redirected more perpendicularly.
- A "pop" can be felt when the needle penetrates the common sheath between the humeral artery and median nerve.
- 6 to 8 mL of local anesthetic solution.

- A catheter can be inserted for a continuous brachial plexus block.

MUSCULOCUTANEOUS

Landmark: Above the median n.

Tips:
- Deeper (1 to 2 cm) into the coracobrachialis muscle just above the median nerve (n.).
- Small nerve, easily blocked; 4 to 5 mL of local anesthetic is usually adequate.

ULNAR

Landmark: Below the median n.

Tips:
- Needle angled 45 degrees posterior.
- 1 to 2 cm deep.
- Sometimes very close to the median n. and partially blocked by the preceding injection.

If you cannot find it, check to see if it is not already blocked.
- *Possible Martin and Gruber anastomosis.*

RADIAL

Landmark: Posterior to the humerus.

Tips:
- At the same level as the ulnar n.
- Needle redirected perpendicular to the skin.
- Nerve is posterior to the humerus (bone contact), 5 to 10 mm deeper.
- Sometimes the nerve can be reached only by doing a slow external rotation of the arm or a more posterior insertion of the needle.

CUTANEOUS BRANCHES

- From the needle insertion point, medial and lateral subcutaneous ring infiltration for the cutaneous nerves of the arm.

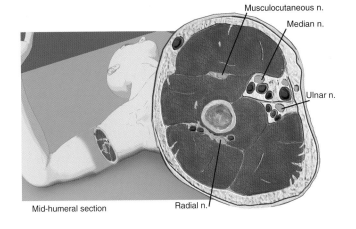

Musculocutaneous n.

Median n.

Ulnar n.

Radial n.

Mid-humeral section

MID-HUMERAL APPROACH

Patient position: Supine, arm rotated externally.

MEDIAN

Landmarks:
- Elbow flexion crease.
- Medial to the brachial artery and biceps tendon.

Tips:
- Tip of the index finger against the medial side of the biceps tendon, above the brachial artery. Needle is inserted medial to the fingertip perpendicular to the skin.
  Nerve will be located at 1 to 2 cm depth.
- Motor response similar to above.

RADIAL

Landmarks:
- Elbow flexion crease.
- Intercondylar fold.
- 1 cm lateral to the biceps tendon.

Tips:
- Tip of the index finger against the lateral side of the biceps tendon.
  Needle is inserted lateral to the fingertip perpendicular to the skin.
- An extension and supination of the forearm will occur when the deep radial branch is stimulated. The deep radial branch innervates the forearm musculature and the posterior part of carpal bones.

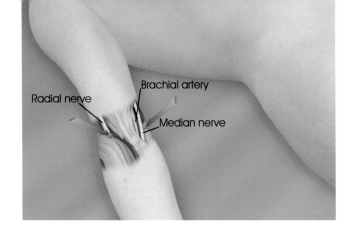

Radial nerve

Brachial artery

Median nerve

RADIAL AND MEDIAN
AT THE ELBOW

ULNAR

Landmarks:
- Ulnar groove.
- With the elbow flexed, the needle is introduced at the apex of a triangle, with the line from the medial epicondyle to the olecranon process as a base.

Tips:
- **DO NOT inject between the medial epicondyle of the humerus and the olecranon process.**
- Motor response similar to above.

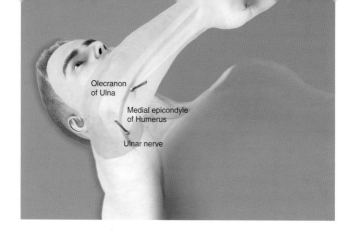

Olecranon
of Ulna

Medial epicondyle
of Humerus

Ulnar nerve

ULNAR AT THE ELBOW

MUSCULOCUTANEOUS

Landmarks: Lateral to the tendon of the biceps.

Tips:
- Below the elbow, the musculocutaneous n. emerges lateral to the tendon of the biceps and descends over the lateral aspect of forearm (lateral cutaneous n. of the forearm). At this level it is a *purely sensory* nerve.
- Subcutaneous infiltration at the level of the elbow crease, under the cephalic vein, from the biceps tendon to the radial head.
- *Neurostimulation (1 msec):* elicits a paresthesia in the musculocutaneous territory.

MEDIAN

Landmarks:
- Lateral to the palmaris longus tendon.
- Medial to the flexor carpi radialis tendon.

Tips:
- Insertion of the needle *5 to 6 cm above the wrist flexion crease.*
  Proximal to the wrist flexion crease, the median n. gives off a palmar cutaneous branch (lateral palmar skin).
- *Median at the wrist is 70% to 80% sensory (anterior) and 20% to 30% motor (posterior).* A needle inserted perpendicular to the skin can elicit paresthesia without motor nerve stimulation. ***Nerve stimulation at 1 msec is used to elicit paraesthesia.***
- Motor response = translation of the thumb.

ULNAR

Landmarks: Below the flexor carpi ulnaris tendon.

Tips:
- Insert needle perpendicular to the skin, below the carpi ulnaris tendon and *4 to 5 cm above the wrist flexion crease.*
- Same motor response as above.
- Interosseous or hypothenor eminence muscles contraction.
- Absence of adduction of the wrist (ulnar inclination of the wrist).

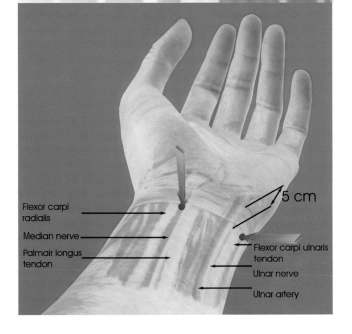

Flexor carpi
radialis

Median nerve

Palmair longus
tendon

5 cm

Flexor carpi ulnaris
tendon

Ulnar nerve

Ulnar artery

MEDIAN AND ULNAR AT THE WRIST

RADIAL

Landmarks: Above the radial artery in the anatomic snuff box.

Tips:
- Subcutaneous infiltration anteriorly and posteriorly at the level of the radial styloid.
- Below the wrist, the radial nerve is purely sensory.

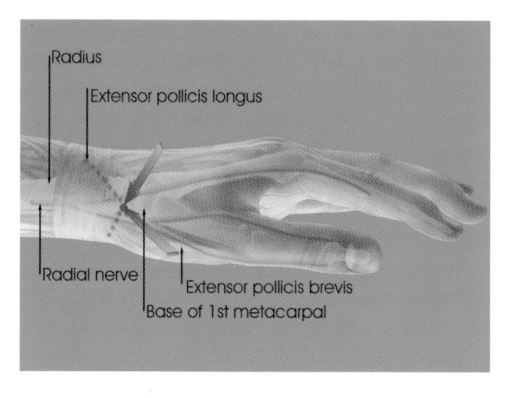

RADIAL AT THE WRIST

FLEXOR DIGITORUM SHEATH BLOCK

Landmarks:
- Metacarpophalangeal (MP) joint of the third digit.
- Flexor tendon.

Tips:
- Surgical block for 2nd, 3rd, and 4th fingers.
- Subcutaneous needle, bevel anterior.
- 45 degrees to the skin until the flexor tendon is reached.
- **A passive flexion of the third finger brings the needle into a vertical position.**
- The needle is slowly withdrawn. The contact with the tendon is lost but the needle is still in the sheath.
- 5 to 8 mL of local anesthetic solution.
- **No epinephrine.**

FLEXOR DIGITORUM SHEATH BLOCK

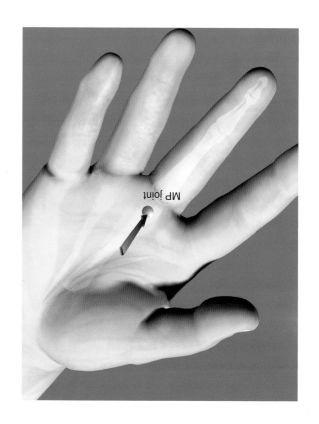

MP joint

Lower Extremity Landmarks

DERMATOMES

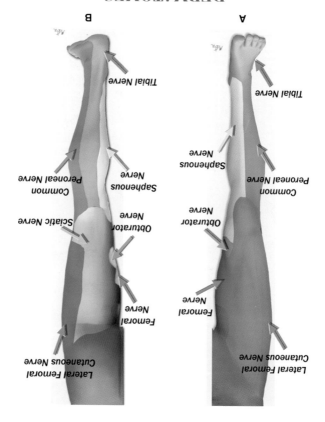

A

Tibial Nerve

Saphenous Nerve

Common Peroneal Nerve

Obturator Nerve

Femoral Nerve

Lateral Femoral Cutaneous Nerve

B

Tibial Nerve

Common Peroneal Nerve

Saphenous Nerve

Sciatic Nerve

Obturator Nerve

Femoral Nerve

Lateral Femoral Cutaneous Nerve

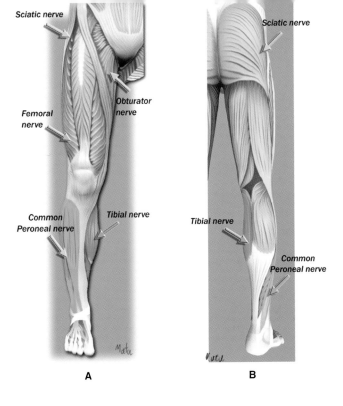

A

B

MYOTOMES

47

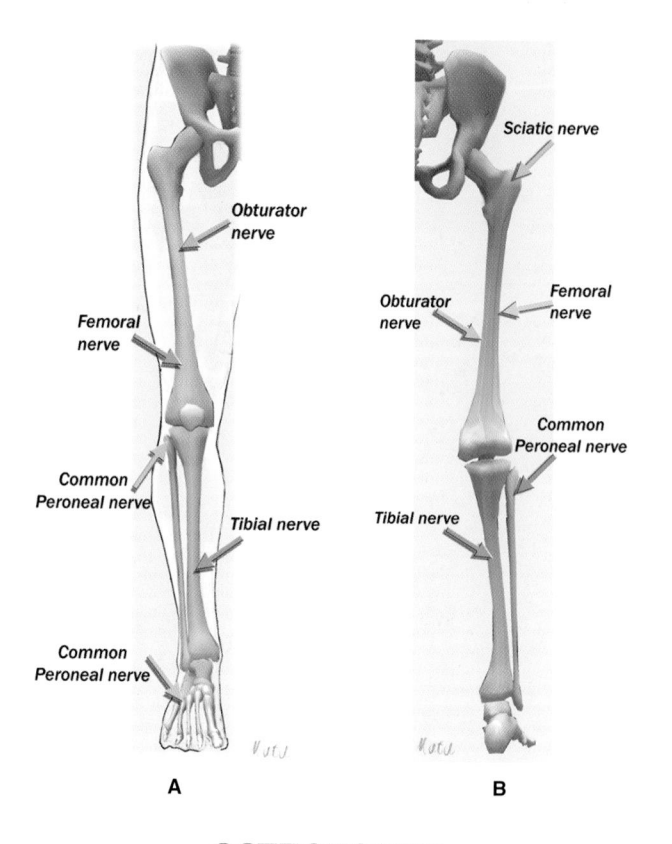

OSTEOTOMES

SCIATIC NERVE

- Inferior division of lumbar L4, L5 and sacral S1, S2, S3 nerves.
- Emerges from the greater sciatic foramen.
- Lies below the piriformis muscle (m.), deep to gluteus maximus m. on the posterior wall of the pelvis.
- Descends between the greater trochanter of the femur and the ischial tuberosity.
- Splits into the common peroneal and tibial nerves. This division may take place at any point between the sacral plexus and the lower third of the thigh.
- *Articular branches arise from the upper part of the nerve and supply the hip joint.*

POSTERIOR FEMORAL CUTANEOUS NERVE

Sacral S1, S2, S3 nerves.

A • Emerges from the pelvis through the greater sciatic foramen below the piriformis.

S • All sensory branches.
• Skin of the perineum.
• Posterior surface of the thighs and legs.

COMMON PERONEAL NERVE

L4, L5, sacral S1, S2 nerves.

A • Winds around the neck of the fibula from posterior to lateral.
• Divides into superficial and deep peroneal nerves.
• The *superficial peroneal nerve* gives innervation to the skin on the dorsum of the foot.
• The *deep peroneal nerve* gives innervation to extensor muscles of the ankle and foot and the skin on first dorsal web space.

• Knee joint and ankle joint (deep peroneal).
• Posterior and lateral aspect of the calf.
• Tarsal and metatarsal joints.
• Dorsum of the foot and toes.

 • Deep peroneal nerve stimulation.
• Dorsiflexion of the foot.
• Eversion.

TIBIAL NERVE

L4, L5, sacral S1, S2, S3 nerves.

 • Passes down in the midline into the fossa between the semitendinosus and biceps femoris m. and lies lateral to the popliteal artery.
• Divides into terminal branches, medial and lateral plantar n., and calcaneal n.
• Sural n. arises in the poplitea fossa and pierces the deep fascia to become subcutaneous.

S
- Knee joint and ankle joint (*tibial n.*).
- Skin on the lower lateral and posterior part of the calf, the lateral part of the foot, and the little toe (*sural n.*).
- Heel and skin of the medial part of the sole (*calcaneal n.*).
- Skin of the sole (*lateral and medial plantar n.*).

N
- Plantar flexion, inversion.
- Flexion of the toes.

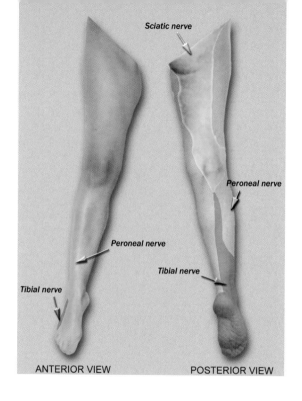

ANTERIOR VIEW   POSTERIOR VIEW

SCIATIC NERVE: DERMATOMES

In relation to the lesser trochanter, they are divided into proximal and distal approaches.

In relation to the surface of the thigh, they are divided into anterior, lateral, and posterior approaches.

PROXIMAL POSTERIOR APPROACHES:
- *Parasacral*
- *Classic*
- *Lithotomy (Raj' approach)*
- *Subgluteal*

PROXIMAL LATERAL APPROACH

PROXIMAL ANTERIOR APPROACH

DISTAL APPROACHES:
- *Lateral popliteal*
- *High posterior popliteal*
- *Classic posterior popliteal*

PROXIMAL POSTERIOR APPROACH

PARASACRAL APPROACH

Patient position: Patient in lateral position, side to be blocked being nondependent, both hips and knees flexed.

Landmarks:
- Line between the posterior superior iliac spine and the ischial tuberosity.
- Insertion point is 6 to 7 cm caudal to the posterior superior iliac spine on this line.

Tips:
- Needle is introduced perpendicular to the skin or at a 30-degree angle in the cranial direction. Upon bone contact (**deep landmark**), the sciatic nerve is located 2 to 3 cm deeper. This bone contact corresponds to the medial part of the

greater sciatic notch of the hip bone. The needle needs to be redirected either caudally or laterally or both.

- A first muscle twitch occurs when the needle is passing through the gluteus muscle. A second, deeper muscle twitch occurs when passing through the piriformis muscle. The nerve is located beneath the piriformis muscle at a depth of 6 to 9 cm.
- If the first distal twitch is a hamstring contraction, deeper advancement of the needle will result in a tibial nerve stimulation (60%) or a combined tibial and common peroneal stimulation (18%).
- At this level, the sciatic nerve is close to internal iliac vessels (sciatic vascular trunk).

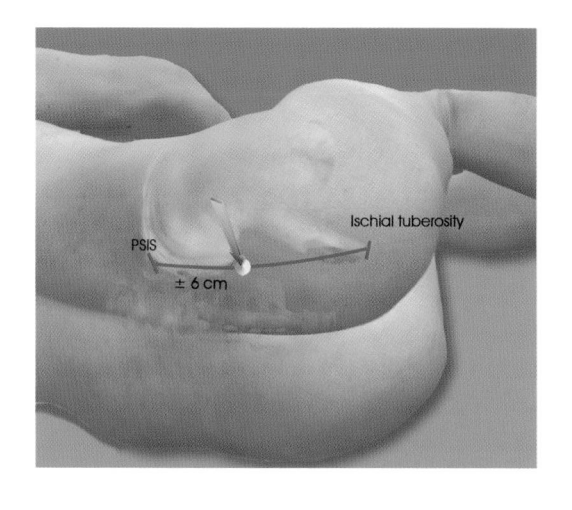

PSIS

± 6 cm

Ischial tuberosity

PARASACRAL APPROACH

CLASSIC POSTERIOR APPROACH

Patient position: Patient in lateral position, side to be blocked being nondependent, with knee and hip flexed (Sim's position).

Landmarks:

- Line between the posterior superior iliac spine and the greater trochanter.
- Perpendicular line is drawn at its midpoint.
- Intersection with a line between the greater trochanter and the sacral hiatus. Or
- 5 cm on a perpendicular line drawn at the midpoint of the line between the posterior superior iliac spine and the greater trochanter.

Tips:

- 4-inch needle.
- Perpendicular to the skin.
- The first contraction is elicited when the needle passes through the gluteus maximus muscle; then a deeper muscular contraction occurs when the needle passes through the piriformis muscle.
- A tibial or peroneal neurostimulation is elicited 1 cm deeper.
- Multistimulation: a dorsiflexion and eversion of the foot (peroneal nerve) means that the needle is stimulating the lateral part of the sciatic nerve.

A tibial n. stimulation will be elicited by
moving the needle medially.

- Bone contact = lateral part of the greater sciatic
  notch of the hip bone. The needle must be redirected medially, caudally, or both.

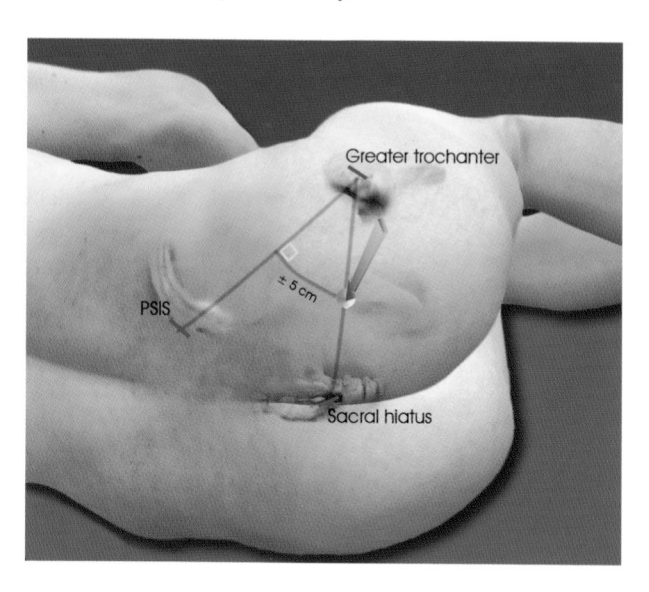

CLASSIC POSTERIOR APPROACH

LITHOTOMY (RAJ' APPROACH)

Patient position: Patient in supine position, an assistant holds the leg to be blocked with the knee and hip flexed.

Landmarks: Midpoint of a line between the greater trochanter and ischial tuberosity.

Tips:
- Needle is introduced perpendicular to the skin.
- Nerve is located at a depth of 5 to 7 cm.
- Stimulation of the tibial or common peroneal nerve (hamstrings may be direct muscle stimulation).

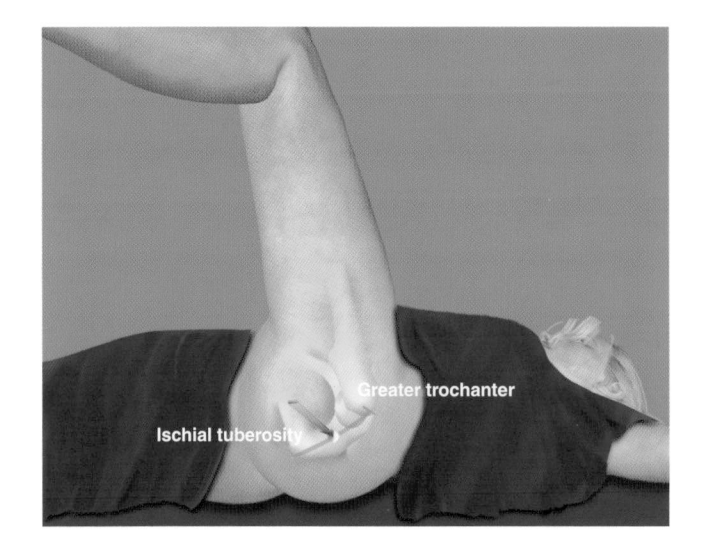

Greater trochanter

Ischial tuberosity

LITHOTOMY (RAJ' APPROACH)

SUBGLUTEAL APPROACH

Patient position: Patient in lateral position, side to be blocked being nondependent, with hip and knee flexed (Sim's position).

Landmarks:
- Line between the greater trochanter and ischial tuberosity.
- 5 to 6 cm caudate on a perpendicular line drawn from its midpoint.

Tips:
- Needle is introduced perpendicular to the skin.
- Nerve is located at a depth of 4 to 6 cm.
- Tibial nerve or common peroneal nerve is stimulated.
- A catheter can be inserted for a continuous sciatic block.

SUBGLUTEAL APPROACH

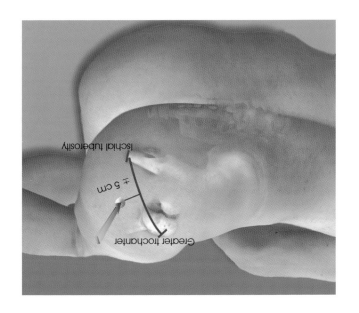

Greater trochanter

± 5 cm

Ischial tuberosity

PROXIMAL LATERAL APPROACH

Patient position: Supine.

Landmarks:
- Great trochanter.
- 2 cm posterior and 2 cm caudal.

Tips:
- 4-inch needle.
- Needle contact with the lateral part of bone.
- 1 to 2 cm deeper.

PROXIMAL ANTERIOR APPROACH

Patient position: Supine.

Landmarks:
- Line between anterior superior iliac spine (ASIS) and superior border of pubic tubercle.
- 8 cm caudate on a perpendicular line drawn from its midpoint.

Tips:
- 4- to 6-inch needle.
- Lateral to the femoral artery (has to be located).
- Femoral nerve can be in the way.
- Needle will contact the lesser trochanter if approach is too proximal. The sciatic nerve runs lateral to the lesser trochanter. To increase the probability of reaching the nerve, internal rotation of the leg is necessary.
- 4 cm below the lesser trochanter, the sciatic nerve runs more medial to the femur.

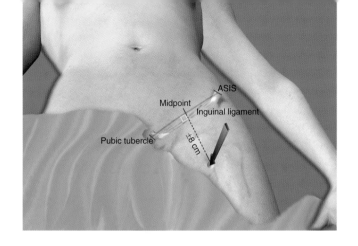

ASIS
Midpoint
Inguinal ligament
Pubic tubercle
±8 cm

PROXIMAL ANTERIOR APPROACH

DISTAL APPROACH

LATERAL POPLITEAL APPROACH

Patient position: Supine, pillow under the knee.

Landmarks:
- Groove between biceps femoris and vastus lateralis muscles (accentuated by asking patient to lift leg).
- 8 to 10 cm above the patella.

Tips:
- Sciatic division in tibial nerve and common peroneal nerve ranges from 4 to 13 cm above popliteal crease.
- 2- or 4-inch needle.
- Needle insertion is perpendicular to the skin, then redirected at a 30-degree angle relative to the horizontal plan.
- The sciatic nerve is deep to the biceps femoris muscle. The first twitch will be a contraction of this muscle.

- A peroneal stimulation is elicited 2 to 3 cm deeper. Internal rotation of the leg may be needed to elicit tibial nerve stimulation.
- When the groove cannot be located, look for contact with the posterior part of the femur. The sciatic nerve is located posteriorly and 1 to 2 cm deeper.
- A catheter can be inserted for a continuous sciatic block.

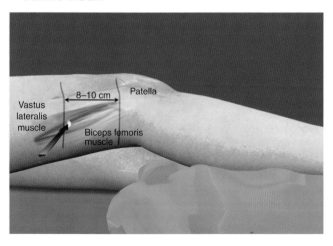

LATERAL POPLITEAL APPROACH

HIGH POSTERIOR POPLITEAL APPROACH

Patient position: Prone, pillow under the foot.

Landmarks:
- Popliteal fossa crease.
- Tendon of the biceps femoris muscle.
- Tendon of the semitendinosus muscle.
- Line along each of the two tendons.
- Lateral border of the intersection of these two lines.

Tips:
- 4-inch needle.
- 30- to 45-degree cranial direction.
- Stimulation of tibial or common peroneal nerve at a depth of 6 to 8 cm.
- A catheter can be inserted for a continuous sciatic block.

CLASSIC POSTERIOR POPLITEAL APPROACH

Patient position: Prone, pillow under the foot.

Landmarks:
- Tendon of the biceps femoris muscle.
- Tendon of the semitendinosus muscle.
- Perpendicular line to the midpopliteal fossa crease.

Tips :
- 2-inch needle.
- Perpendicular to the skin.
- 5 to 7 cm in the cephalad direction of the perpendicular line. Needle is inserted lateral to this point.
- Tibial nerve stimulation.
- Common peroneal nerve is 1 cm lateral to the tibial nerve.

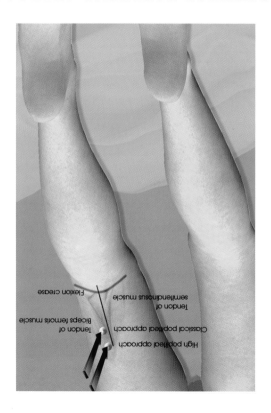

High popliteal approach

Classical popliteal approach

Tendon of
biceps femoris muscle

Tendon of
semitendinosus muscle

Flexion crease

LUMBAR NERVES

- Ventral roots of the first 4 lumbar nerves.
- Lumbar plexus lies within the psoas muscle, anterior to the transverse processes of the L2-L5 vertebrae.

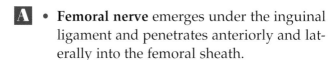

- **Femoral nerve** emerges under the inguinal ligament and penetrates anteriorly and laterally into the femoral sheath.
- **Saphenous nerve** emerges posterior to the sartorius muscle and anterior to gracilis muscle to continue with the long saphenous vein.
- **Obturator nerve** emerges from the obturator foramen and separates into anterior and posterior divisions, which straddle the adductor brevis muscle.
- **Lateral femoral cutaneous nerve** emerges lateral to the psoas muscle below the iliac crest and penetrates the iguinal ligament

at its attachment to pass into the subcutaneous tissue of the lateral thigh.

S • Hip joint (femoral + obturator n.) and femur.
• Knee joint (femoral + obturator n.).
• Medial aspect of the calf and medial forefoot (saphenous n.).

N • Femoral n. = contraction of quadriceps m. (vastus intermedius) with an upward movement of the patella.
• Obturator n. = contraction of the adductor magnus m. (adductor brevis and adductor longus).
• Lateral femoral cutaneous n. = purely sensory.

A Anatomy **S** Surgical field **N** Neurostimulation

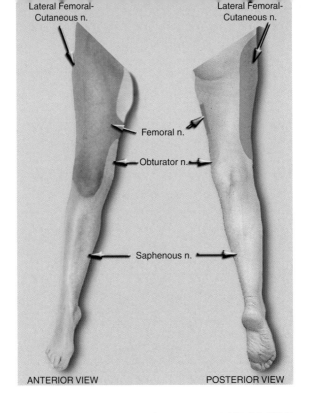

Lateral Femoral-
Cutaneous n.

Lateral Femoral-
Cutaneous n.

Femoral n.

Obturator n.

Saphenous n.

ANTERIOR VIEW

POSTERIOR VIEW

LUMBAR NERVES: DERMATOMES

POSTERIOR APPROACH
(LUMBAR PLEXUS BLOCK)

Patient position: Patient in lateral position, side to be blocked nondependent.

Landmarks:
- Highest point on iliac crest (HPIC).
- Vertebral spine on the midline.
- Posterior superior iliac spine (PSIS).
- Line from the PSIS, parallel to the midline.
- Line from the HPIC to the vertebral spine.
- Puncture point can be at the intersection of these two lines or at 4 cm from the midline.

Tips:
- 4-inch needle.
- Perpendicular to the skin or slightly directed medially if puncture point at the intersection of the two lines.

- After a contact with the transverse process of L4 at 4 to 6 cm (deep landmark), walk the needle off the transverse process cranially or caudally (angle between 30 and 45 degrees).
- The distance from the skin to the transverse process depends on the patient's size. The distance between the transverse process and the plexus is **never more than 2 cm**. A stimulation of the femoral nerve inducing a contraction of the quadriceps should be elicited **1 or 2 cm deeper.**
- Twitching of the hamstring muscles or movement of the foot results from stimulation of a sciatic nerve root. The needle is inserted too caudally and must be redirected to walk off the transverse process cranially.
- A medial contraction of the thigh can be related to an adductor muscle contraction by stimulation of the obturator nerve. The needle must be redirected laterally in order to induce a quadriceps contraction.
- A stimulation with a current intensity below 0.5 mA is not necessary (0.5 to 1 mA is adequate).

- A catheter can be inserted for a continuous femoral block.
- Blood pressure should be monitored closely because of **a possible epidural or subarachnoid injection.**
- A test dose (3 to 5 mL) and a fragmented injection (10 mL/30 sec) of the mixture are essential when a lumbar plexus block is being performed.

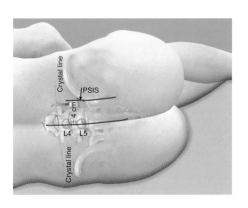

POSTERIOR APPROACH (LUMBAR PLEXUS BLOCK)

ANTERIOR APPROACH
(FEMORAL BLOCK)

Patient position: Supine.

Landmarks:
- Line between ASIS and pubic tubercle (PT).
- Parallel line at the inguinal crease.
- 1 cm lateral to the femoral artery pulse.

Tips:
- If the femoral artery pulse cannot be felt, the puncture point will be approximately **1 cm lateral to a point located 5 cm caudally on a perpendicular line at the midpoint of the line ASIS–PT.**
- A contraction of the vastus medialis indicates a medial and anterior approach of the nerve.
- To obtain a contraction of the vastus intermedius (upward movement of the patella), the needle is directed posterior and laterally.

- Single stimulation = the total dose of local anesthetic is injected when contraction of the vastus intermedius is elicited.
- Multistimulation = injections of 5 to 7 mL local anesthetic, respectively, when a contraction of the vastus medialis, vastus intermedius, and vastus lateralis is elicited.
- Distal pressure and large volume can procure a 3-in-1 block (the obturator nerve is missed most of the time).
- For surgeries below the knee, a saphenous nerve block can be obtained when a vastus medialis contraction is elicited.
- A catheter can be inserted for a continuous femoral block.

ANTERIOR APPROACH (FEMORAL BLOCK)

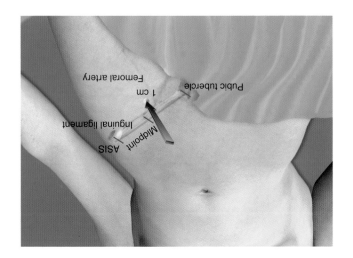

ANTERIOR APPROACH
(FASCIA ILIACA APPROACH)

Patient position: Supine.

Landmarks:
- Line between ASIS and pubic tubercle.
- Divide the line into three parts.
- Insert needle 2 cm below this line at its lateral third.

Tips:
- Tuohy or B-bevel needle.
- Perpendicular to the skin.
- First "pop" and second pop occur when the needle passes through the fascia lata and the fascia iliaca, respectively (occasionally only one pop is obtained).
- A catheter can be inserted for a continuous femoral block.

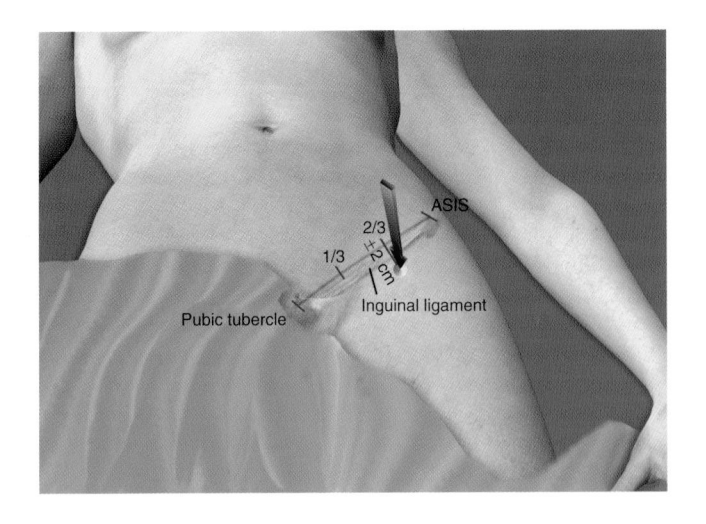

ANTERIOR APPROACH
(FASCIA ILIACA APPROACH)

OBTURATOR NERVE BLOCK (CLASSIC APPROACH)

Patient position: Supine, leg slightly abducted.

Landmarks:
- Pubic tubercle.
- 2 cm lateral and 2 cm caudal.

Tips:
- 2-inch needle.
- Insert perpendicular to the skin, then at a 30- to 40-degree angle in the cranial direction.
- 3- to 4-cm depth (obturator canal).
- 5 mL of local anesthetic.
- *Obturator nerve block is assessed by seeking for adductor muscle weakness.*

OBTURATOR NERVE BLOCK
(DISTAL APPROACH)

Patient position: Supine, leg slightly abducted.

Landmarks:
- Line between ASIS and pubic tubercle.
- Midpoint of a parallel line between femoral artery and medial border of adductor longus at inguinal crease.

Tips:
- Obturator n. is medial to the femoral vein, below the pectineus m. and divides into anterior and posterior branches, which straddle the adductor brevis muscle.
- 2-inch needle.
- 30-degree angle in cranial direction.
- 5 mL of local anesthetic when a contraction of the adductor brevis occurs and an additional 5 mL when a contraction of the adductor longus (deeper) is elicited.

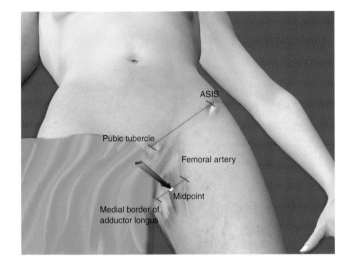

ASIS

Pubic tubercle

Femoral artery

Midpoint

Medial border of
adductor longus

OBTURATOR NERVE BLOCK
(DISTAL APPROACH)

LATERAL FEMORAL CUTANEOUS NERVE BLOCK

Patient position: Supine.

Landmarks:
- ASIS.
- 2 cm caudal and 2 cm medial.

Tips:
- Sensory nerve.
- Paresthesia can be elicited using a 1-msec impulse.

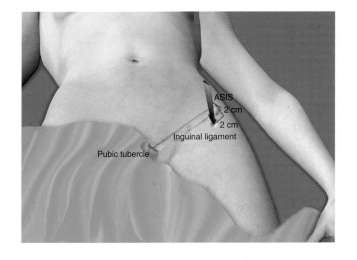

LATERAL FEMORAL CUTANEOUS NERVE BLOCK

SAPHENOUS NERVE BLOCK

Patient position: Supine.

Landmarks:
- Head of the tibia.
- Femoral artery.
- Sartorius muscle.

Tips:
- Sensory nerve.
- Medial subcutaneous infiltration advancing deeper as the needle approaches the gastrocnemius muscle between **the tibial tuberosity and the internal gastrocnemius muscle** (3 cm deep).
  Or
- Femoral neck block (stimulation of the vastus medialis m.).
  Or

- Transsartorial approach: **sartorius muscle** above the medial side of the patella. The needle is inserted at a 45-degree angle posterior to the sartorius muscle.
- Paresthesia can be elicited using a 1-msec impulse.
- 10 mL of local anesthetic.

ANKLE BLOCK

Patient position: Supine.

Posterior tibial nerve

Landmarks:
- Posterior tibial artery.
- Medial malleolus.

Tips:
- 25-gauge or 1-inch needle for possible neurostimulation.
- Injection of 5 mL of local anesthetic posterior to the artery and anterior to the Achilles tendon at the level of the medial malleolus.
- Neurostimulation = flexion of the toes.
- No epinephrine.

Deep peroneal (fibular) nerve

Landmarks:
- Ankle joint.
- Extensor hallucinis longus tendon.
- Anterior tibial artery.

Tips:
- 25-gauge needle.
- Injection of 5 mL of local anesthetic medial to the artery and lateral to the extensor hallucinis longus tendon at the level of the ankle flexion crease.
- No epinephrine.

Sural and superficial peroneal (fibular) nerves
Saphenous nerve (branch of the femoral nerve)

Landmarks:
- Achilles tendon.
- Lateral malleolus.
- Medial malleolus.

Tips:
- 25-gauge needle.
- Subcutaneous ring injection of 10 mL of local anesthetic. One injection from the superior border of the lateral malleolus to the lateral aspect of the Achilles tendon (sural nerve) and one injection from the superior border of the lateral malleolus to the posterosuperior aspect of the medial malleolus (superficial peroneal nerve and saphenous nerve).
- No epinephrine.

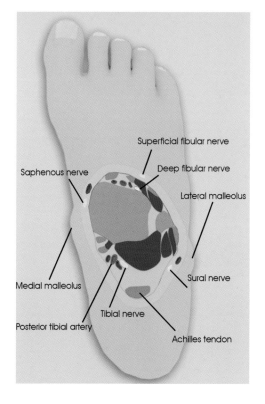

Superficial fibular nerve

Deep fibular nerve

Saphenous nerve

Lateral malleolus

Medial malleolus

Sural nerve

Posterior tibial artery

Tibial nerve

Achilles tendon

ANKLE BLOCK